Contents

Introduction

Fitness Industry is a huge industry and with more people getting conscious about their health it is growing at a tremendous rate, unfortunately some people in the industry spread false information and myths in order to sell their products .This false information is harmful to beginners who really want to make a changes to their physique .Not only these beginners make no progress due to being misinformed but they eventually get discouraged and quit ,thinking that achieving their dream physique is impossible.

My intention with writing this book is to provide the correct information required to get to your dream physique.

Another fact here is that people have made very simple things very complicated .Let me tell you about the 80-20 Rule, Your 80% results come from 20% of the work you do. It is true in reverse where 80% of the work you do makes up for only 20% of your results .Simple things have been so overcomplicated for beginners and their focus has been diverted from the 20% work that gives 80% result to the 80% work that gives only about 20% of the results. This is the reason sometimes people think that building your dream physique is hard and very complicated, and they ultimately quit because they only get little to no result for the hard work they did. That's because they did hard work in the wrong place.

This isn't going to be a 200 page book that just tells you the stuffs that's not going to help you, or complicate things for you ,instead its going to be book that teaches you the fundamentals of bodybuilding and diet so that you can attain the physique you always wanted to have by yourself ,explained in a simple and understandable language.

You might find a lot of sample workouts and diets online ,some paid and some free ,you might be someone who has tried those diets and workouts and didn't get any result ,the reason isn't that ,that these diets or workouts don't work ,it is, just that, these diets and workouts doesn't work for you.

Remember everybody is different , Every-Body is different. What works for someone might not work for you ,what works for you might not work for someone else. This book will solve that problem by teaching you the **Fundamentals of Bodybuilding**, so you can create your own workouts and diet plan ,that works for you. The best way will always be trial and error in my opinion ,test what has been taught in this book and see for yourself, what works for you and what doesn't .

After completing this book you should be able to make your own Diet and Workout Plan.

In this book various figures and ranges have been mentioned most of them are just approximate numbers as it is really hard/nearly impossible to be 100% accurate but these numbers are something that works for most people ,and will really help beginners ,who have no idea what to do. For most ranges suggested you can take somewhat of the middle of the ranges in most cases. These numbers are what i used on myself and my clients to see amazing results.

 If you apply the Principles in this book and work hard you can achieve your dream physique. Remember ,Bodybuilding is a Science but it is also a Mindset, if you are persistent and consistent you will one day reach your goals.

All the Best, for your Fitness Journey!

Calories

Calories are the most important factor ,when it comes to gaining weight or losing weight. The calories in a food is the amount of Potential Energy that food has. Our body uses these calories to fuel our various body functions. The Calorie requirement differs from individual to individual. Our bodies need certain amount of these calories to maintain its current weight also known as the **Maintenance Calories** ,If you eat in a **Caloric Surplus** ,that is ,eating more calories than your Maintenance Calories then the extra calories are used for building muscles or are stored as fat ,**resulting in Weight Gain**. And when you eat in a **Caloric Deficit**, that is ,eating less calories than your Maintenance Calories you will **Lose Weight** .

Now the question arises that what are your Maintenance Calories ?

Before calculating Maintenance calories you should know that the Maintenance Calories is not static it changes due to various variables like your activity level ,age ,your training intensity etc. So it is really hard to measure them exactly but there are some ways by which you can get a good estimation of your maintenance calories.

To find your maintenance calories you can use the **Calorie Calculators** available online or you can find your approximate **Maintenance Calories by using this simple formula:-**

Maintenance Calories = Your Bodyweight in Lbs. X 14-16

Example:- 150 lbs. X 14-16 = 2100-2400 Calories

Now what you have got is a Range of Maintenance calories (2100-2400 Calories) you can now use somewhat middle of this Range (let's say, 2250 Calories) and use it as a Starting Point. Consume these calories for about 2-3 weeks and measure your weight changes. The thing with measuring your progress by using Weight Machine is that ,your weight fluctuates everyday. Some days you might weigh a little less whereas some other days you might weigh a little more,so what you have to do is, use your Average Weekly weight of 2-4 weeks and compare them.If your average weekly weight does not change by a lot that means you are eating at your Maintenance. If its decreasing continuously, it means you need to eat slightly more and if its increasing it means you have to eat a little less.

That 2250 Calories is the approximate amount of calories you need to eat each day to maintain your weight.

Now if you want to gain weight you have to eat more calories **(Caloric Surplus)** and if you want to lose weight you will have to eat less calories than your maintenance calories **(Calorie Deficit).**

There are a lot of Fad Diets out there, that tells you if you want to lose weight ,eat this eat that, don't eat this don't eat that, most of them don't work but the ones that do follows this simple **Principle of Calories in vs Calories out**.

Behind the curtain all those diets that works and allows you to lose fat puts you in a **Calorie Deficit**. Now i am not against any of those diets, you can try them if you want, but i feel that some of them are overly restrictive, and really hard to sustain over long period of time. If its too restrictive you will give upon it soon before you make any significant progress.

Bodybuilding is a Marathon not a Sprint .When choosing a diet choose what you can sustain over a long period of time, and something that fits your lifestyle so you don't feel being left out of things. As long as you eat in a deficit you will lose weight .Stop trying to overcomplicate it.

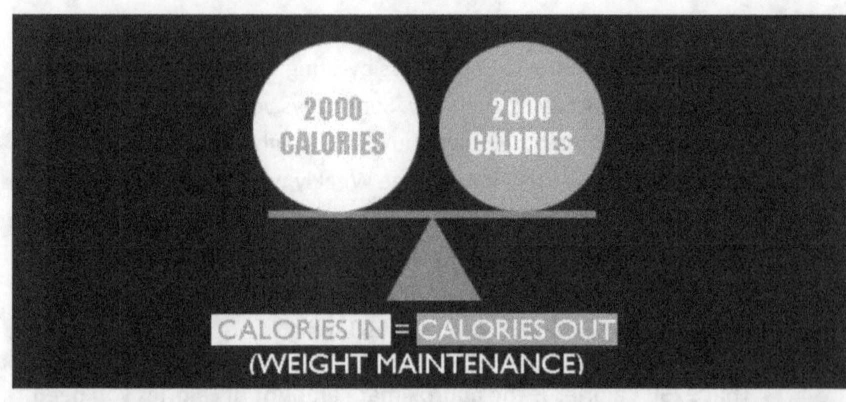

2000 CALORIES
2000 CALORIES
CALORIES IN = CALORIES OUT
(WEIGHT MAINTENANCE)

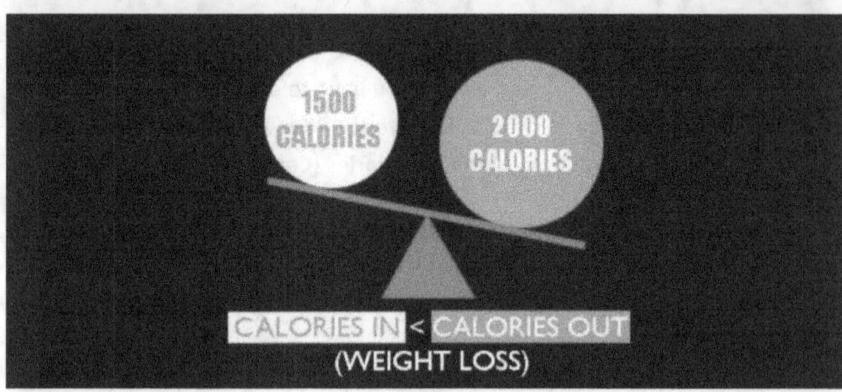

1500 CALORIES
2000 CALORIES
CALORIES IN < CALORIES OUT
(WEIGHT LOSS)

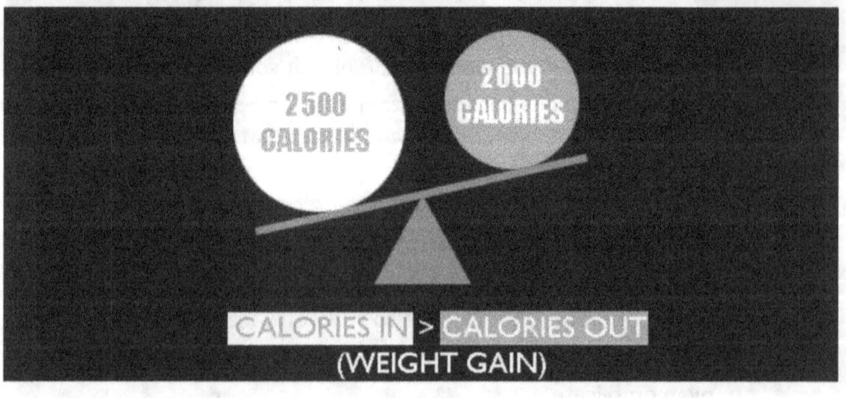

2500 CALORIES
2000 CALORIES
CALORIES IN > CALORIES OUT
(WEIGHT GAIN)

Macros

Since now you know the basics about Calories, let's move on to the other crucial concept that is our **Macros.**

The food we eat has got Macros (Macronutrient) in it. Macros are the nutrients that our body needs for energy and to maintain body structure and system.

There are 3 Macronutrients:-

1) Protein (4 Calories/gram)

Protein are the essential amino acids that helps in the recovery and muscle growth of your body. Each gram of Protein contains 4 calories in it. A lot of times people will tell you to eat as much protein as you humanly can but it is not very accurate .Generally , you need to eat just 0.8-1 gm protein/lbs. of your bodyweight. If you are slightly obese/have bodyfat percentage >20% you can use your **Lean Body Mass** instead of body weight.

Lean Body Mass = Your Total Weight in Lbs. X (100% – Your Bodyfat %)

Example:- 250 Lbs. X (100% – 30% (Bodyfat percentage)) = 175 Lbs.

Some great sources of Protein are- Eggs ,Chicken ,Milk ,Beans ,Lentils etc.

2) Carbohydrates (4 Calories/gram)

Carbs are our body's primary energy source that are used as fuel by our brain and muscles. Each gram of carb contains 4 calories in it.

Some great sources of Carbs are-Oats ,Rice ,Pasta ,Banana ,Potatoes etc.

3) Fats (9 calories/gram)

Many people consider fat as a bad thing and avoid eating them whenever possible, people think that eating fat will make them fat, which is not accurate, eating in a Calorie Surplus makes people gain weight. Fat is essential for optimal hormonal environment in our body and absorption of various vitamins and nutrients in our body. Some great sources of Fat are-Olive oil, Nuts, Egg Yolk, cold water fish etc.

How to set up your Diet?

Since you now know about Calories and Macros , let's get started with how to set up **Your Own Personalised Diet Plan.**

We will start with estimating your Maintenance Calories .For the sake of understanding we will assume that your Weight is 150 lbs so your maintenance calories will be ~2250 **calories.**

Now that we know the calories required to maintain your weight ,Now we will see how Your Macros should look like.

> **Protein:- 150 gm (1 gm/Lbs. Of Bodyweight) :- 600 calories**
> **(150 gm Protein X 4 calories/gm)**

This means that we will consume 600 Calories from protein.

Now we got 1650 Calories remaining (2250 - 600 Calories) you can consume those from fats and carbs its your choice.

But still i would suggest to not cut out all carb or all fats. You have to consume both as both are essential. I would say, take at least 20-35% of your maintenance calories from fats.

That would mean 2250 X 25 % = 562 calories (562 Calories ÷ 9 Calories (As fat has 9 Calories/gm))= 62 gm approx

Now that we got 600 calories from 150gm protein, and 562 calories from 62gm fat, we got 1088 calories remaining ,out of total 2250 Calories, Now we will consume the remaining 1088 Calories from carbs, which will come to about 272gm of carbs (1088 calories ÷ 4 (As Carbs has 4 Calories/gm)).

So your macro split for 2250 calories at Bodyweight of 150 Lbs would look like:-

- ➢ **Protein -150 gm**
- ➢ **Carbs - 272 gm**
- ➢ **Fats - 62 gm**

Now that you know how to calculate the calories and macros lets know how to approach **Bulking** and **Cutting.**

How to decide whether to Bulk or Cut?

If you have more than 15-25% Body fat you might want to cut and if you have less than 10% Body fat you might want to bulk. This again depends on your goals and is really your choice. In simple words, If you are at higher fat percentage than what you want to be at then you should Cut and if you are at a lower fat percentage than what you want to have, you should Bulk. There might be a case where people might be Skinny Fat, a case where people are both skinny and fat, meaning they might have a lot of fat around their waist and have completely skinny legs or arms. There are a lot of approaches to deal with it but without overcomplicating it the simplest one, i would recommend , is to Cut first, while properly training, and then when you get to your desired body fat level you can start Bulking your way up to your dream body.

How to count Calories and Macros?

To count your calories and macros you can use apps like myfitnesspal that tells you about the amount of calories in your food along with its macros. You can simply select the food that you are eating and its quantity and you will get an estimate of its calories and macros.

Bulking

If you are someone that just want to gain weight no matter if its fat or muscle then you can eat in a larger surplus (Dirty Bulk), than someone who is looking to gain mostly muscle and a little to no fat (Clean Bulk).Let me tell you this, muscle building is a really slow process but it is worth it. A good number if you ask me if you have amazing genetics and when everything like your Diet, Training, Recovery is perfect, is 0.5-2 lbs. a month as a Beginner ,also you won't grow the muscle at the same rate as you do as a beginner. As you keep on lifting, rate at which you gain muscle will eventually decrease.

As Everybody has a natural limit to gain muscles or else people would just keep on lifting and gaining muscles forever and be looking like Arnold Naturally.

Although 0.5-1 Lbs is a small number but think of it like this, that over a period of 1 year you will gain 6-12 Lbs. of lean muscle mass. And that is going to bring massive changes to your Physique.

Lean Bulking

Assuming that your goal is to Gain most amount of muscles possible without gaining a lot of fat i will suggest you to go with Clean Bulking.

It takes approx. 1000 calories to build 1 lbs. of Muscle. Assuming we gain 1 Lbs of Muscle each month it will take us at least ~33 calories each day extra to build muscles. Which is a really low surplus. So for clean bulking we can try eating 100-200 calories extra and see how our body reacts. If you gain too much, the surplus might be too high.

The benefit of clean bulking over Dirty Bulking (Where the surplus is high that is, >300 calories) is that we get to maintain a decent shape/Bodyfat percentage throughout the muscle building phase and also at the end we don't gain a lot of unnecessary fat, so we don't have to go through the long cutting phase to get into the Shape/Bodyfat we desired.

Diet for Bulking

Bulking Calories = Maintenance calories + 100 to 200 Calories (Start from the lower range)

Macros for Bulking

- ➢ **Protein**:- 0.8 to 1 gm/Lbs. Of Bodyweight
- ➢ **Fats**:- 25 to 35 % Of the Total Calories should come from Fats
- ➢ **Carbs**:- Consume Carbs for the Remaining Calories

Example:- Let's say your Bodyweight is 150 lbs and your maintenance is 2250 Calories for Bulking your calories should be 2350 Calories (2250 Calories + 100 Calories)

- ➢ **Protein**:- 150 gm (1gm/lbs. Of your Bodyweight):- 600 calories (150 gm Protein X 4 calories/gm)
- ➢ **Fats** :- 25 to 35% of Total Calories :- 587 Calories (2350 Calories X 25 %) :- 587 Calories ÷ 9 = 65 gm Fat
- ➢ **Carbs** :- 2350 Calories – 600 calories from protein – 587 Calories from Fat :- 1163 calories ÷ 4 = 290 gm Carbs

Tip:- When bulking you can go with higher range of fat, as fat is calorie dense (9 Calories/gm as compared to 4 Calories/gm of Carbs and Protein) and will help you consume extra calories more easily.

Cutting

Before we get into this its important for you to know that 1lbs of fat contains about 3500 Calories (approx).So if in a week you will eat 500 calories more than your maintenance you will gain 1 lbs of fat and if you will eat 500 calories less per day (i.e. Maintenance calories – 500 calories),for a week you will lose 1lbs of fat. Getting in a Calorie Deficit is crucial for fat loss. You can get into deficit by either consuming less calories or by burning more calories. I would suggest to start with eating less and when you get to the point where you can't eat any less than what you are already eating ,you can start doing some cardio to burn some more calories. With Cutting, your main goal will not be just to lose fat but also to preserve your hard earned muscles.

For preserving the most amount of Muscles gained we have to ensure your Calorie Deficit is not too large based on your goals. A large calorie deficit is really hard to sustain over a period of time so its better to start with a smaller deficit so that it is sustainable for longer period of time and fits your lifestyle better.

A Small Calorie deficit over a longer period of time is better than Large Deficit for short period,that is really hard to sustain.

How much Weight should you Lose?

0.5% to 1.5% of Bodyweight/Week ,is a healthy amount of weight to lose, depending on your bodyfat levels. In starting , start with 1.5% as you have a lot more fat to lose and eventually lower it down to 0.5% as it becomes harder to diet. In the starting week you might lose more weight ,which might be caused due to lower water retention but after that if you are still losing weight very fast you might want to up your calories a little bit.

What should be the size of the Deficit?

Let's say that you weigh 200 lbs and you want to lose 1% of that, so that will be 2 Lbs. Per week.

Since 1 Lbs. Of fat has 3500 Calories you will need to eat 7000 Calories (2 lbs X 3500 Calories) Less per week to lose 2 Lbs. Of fat, which will come to about 1000 Calorie deficit Per day.

Preserving Muscles during Cutting

During Cutting, as you are in a deficit you might lose some strength and some muscle mass, along with fat. In order to Preserve your hard earned muscles make sure you:-

> **Eat Protein**

During Cut make sure you are eating enough protein (0.8 – 1 gm/Lbs. Of your Bodyweight).Protein is crucial not just to build muscles but to also Preserve muscles. You can also up your Protein during the cut if you want to 1-1.3 gm/Lbs. Of your bodyweight, as it is most satiating Macronutrient, and will make you feel more full when you are in a deficit and will also ensure muscle preservation .

> **Training properly while Cutting**

Your training doesn't have to change a lot. Although you might lose some strength during your cut , which is normal, but make sure you try to lift almost the same amount of weight as you used to before. If your rep range falls to below 6-8 reps, with the weight you used to do 10-12 reps with, lower the weight slightly and adjust your training according to the concepts explained in the **Training** chapter later.

Diet for Cutting

Calories for Cutting = Maintenance calories - 300 to 1000 Calories (Depends on your goals)

Macros for Cutting

- ➢ **Protein**:- 1 to 1.3 gm/Lbs. Of Bodyweight
- ➢ **Fats**:- 20 to 30% Of the total Calories should come from Fat
- ➢ **Carbs**:- Consume Carbs for the Remaining Calories

Example:- Let's say your Bodyweight is 150 lbs and your maintenance is 2250 Calories for Cutting your calories should be:-

Calories during Cutting :- Maintenance calories – The amount of calories you should eat less each day to lose weight at your desired Rate .

How to find The amount of calories you should eat less each day to lose weight at your desired Rate?

Let's say you want to lose 0.5 % of your body weight per week that would be 0.75 lbs/week. (150 Lbs X 0.5%)

Now since a pound of fat is made up of ~3500 calories you will need to eat 2625 calories (0.75 Lbs. X 3500 calories) less per week, that would come to about 375 calories per day (2625 Calories ÷ 7 Days).

Let's start with eating 400 calories less each day in the starting just to stay at the safer side.

Calories for cutting will be = 1850 Calories (2250 Calories – 400 Calories)

- ➢ **Protein**:-150 gm (1.2 gm/lbs. Of your Bodyweight):- 720 calories(180 gm Protein X 4 calories/gm)
- ➢ **Fats** :- 25 to 35% of Total Calories :- 463 Calories (1850 Calories X 25 %) :- 463 Calories ÷ 9 (Fat has 9 Calories/gm) = 51 gm Fat
- ➢ **Carbs** :- 1850 Calories – 720 calories from Protein – 463 Calories from Fat :- 667 calories ÷ 4(Carbs has 4 Calories/gm) = 166 gm Carbs

The diet has higher amount of Protein as compared to Bulking one as Protein is more satiating and helps build and preserve muscle during the cut, you can eat 1gm/Lbs. Of Your Bodyweight, if you want to, also the percentage of calories that comes from fat is lower of the range here as fat is calorie dense (9 calories/gm of Fat).

Tips For Cutting

Remember our weight changes every day and even throughout the day. Some day you might weigh a little more and some days a little less. Hence you should focus on average weekly weight, and use it for comparison over weeks to actually track your progress. Also make sure you measure your weight at the same time, each day, preferably after you poop, and at the beginning of your day. As long as you are losing weight gradually over a period of time, the daily fluctuations does not matter.

You can also use body measurements to keep a good track your progress over a period of time.

Also instead of focusing on your daily calories you can focus on your **Average Weekly Calories**, as it is the Average Weekly Calories that matters .

Suppose your weekly Maintenance Calories is 2500 and in order to lose weight you have to eat an average of 500 calories less each day, So you can follow any of the two approaches:-

➢ **Either you can eat 2000 calories everyday keeping the weekly average to 2000 Calories**

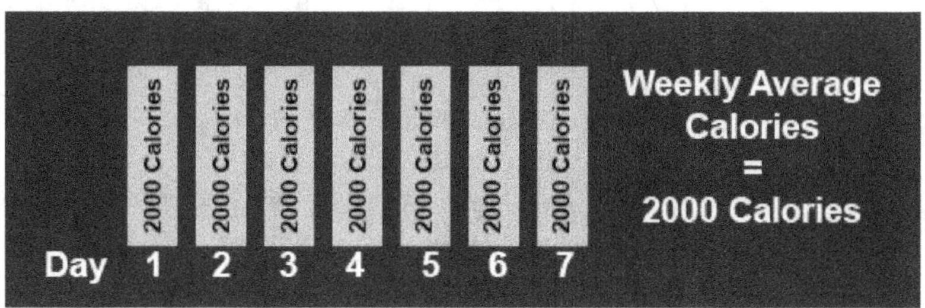

➢ **Or you can eat More calories on some days and a little bit less on the others , but keeping your Weekly Average Calories same to 2000 Calories.**

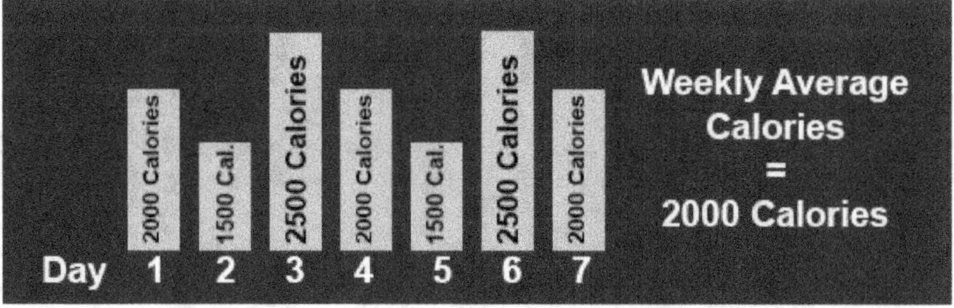

The second approach or **The Calorie Cycling** approach is great while cutting as it allows you to eat slightly more on the days before your workout so that you have energy to perform your workout the next day. This also makes dieting less boring and more sustainable.

How to get Abs?

A lot of people try to lose weight from specific places but the truth is that you can't spot reduce fat. Where the fat is stored in your body is genetically determined. Sometimes the places you gain the fat the fastest are the last places from where you lose fat. Since you can't spot reduce fat you should focus on the calorie deficit for a longer period of time and eventually you will lose fat from those places too.

So, doing Abs exercises will not spot reduce your Belly fat .

We all have abs but they are covered with a layer of fat. Doing abs exercises you will grow your abs ,but you won't be able to see those abs unless you remove the layer of fat covering them.

 It is true that abs are made in the gym where you train them, but are revealed in the kitchen as you diet down to lose the fat covering them.

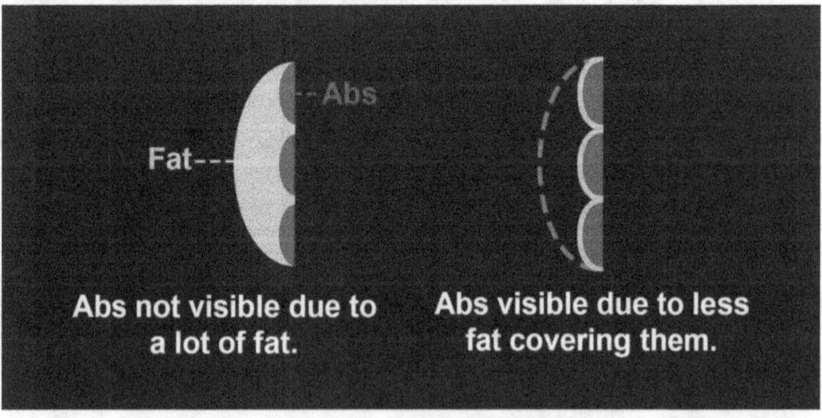

Summarising Dieting

Saying it again if you will eat in a **Caloric Surplus** you will **Gain Weight** and if you eat in a **Caloric Deficit** you will **Lose Weight**. Its just that simple. A lot of times people think they can't gain weight, that's because they eat less their maintenance and they overestimate the food that they eat whereas the people complaining they can't lose weight eat at or below their Maintenance and underestimate the calories that they eat.

This covers our nutrition aspect of the Bodybuilding.Nutrition is considered to give 70% of the results and the rest 30% is covered by Proper Training and Recovery to achieve your Dream Physique. This doesn't make one more important than other, You have to give your 100% in both dieting and Training to get 100% results.

How do Muscles Grow ?

Simplifying the complicated process muscles size increases as we provide it with a stimulus which in case is going to be our Resistance Training/lifting weights, this stimulus causes damages to our muscle fibers. When we provide our body with adequate fuel and Rest, it regenerates the damaged muscles and grows the muscles, leading to muscle growth.(Recovery)

TRAINING

There is no specific amount of set, reps, order of exercises or amount of weight that you have to use to get the maximum results. You can't just copy your favourite bodybuilder's workout routine and expect the same results. Every individual is different and different things work for each individual. However, if you understand the basic fundamentals of training you will be able to pick out the best from amongst the various alternatives available to you.

By understanding the fundamentals you will be able to draw up your own tailored workout plan with the weight, sets and reps best for you.

> - **Reps**- Number of times you lift a weight. For Example:- You take a Dumbbell and do 12 Repetitions with it, these repetitions are called Reps.
> - **Sets**- A group of Repetition is called a set. The 12 reps you did in the above example would be considered as one Set.

What Exercises should you do?

There are two types of exercises or movements namely the **Compound Movements** and the **Isolation Movements.**

Compound Movements v/s Isolation Movements

Compound Movements are the movements that involves various muscle group during an exercise for example :- **Deadlifts** (Involves back,legs etc.), **Squats** (Involves core, legs, glutes), **Bench Press** (Involves chest, triceps), **Pullup/Chin up** (Involves biceps, back), **Dips** (Involves chest, triceps), **Overhead Press** (Involves shoulders, triceps) on the other hand **Isolation Movements** are those that only involves a a single muscle group during an exercise, for example :-**Bicep Curl** (Involves bicep), **Chest Fly** (Involves chest).Most beginners focus on isolation movements and almost completely ignore the Compound Movements. The opposite of what they should be doing.

About ~80% of your workout should consist of Compound Movements and the rest ~20% should consist of the Isolation Movements. As a lifter you should start by doing Compound Movements in the starting of the workout and then move to Isolation Movements at the end of your workout to work on the Glamour muscles(Biceps, Shoulders, Triceps etc.).

TIP:-The Compound movements allows you to lift heavier weights, so maintaining a proper form is crucial, so you don't end up hurting yourself. When learning a compound movement you can start with mastering the Form first, with an empty bar and practice your form. When your feel that your form is correct, then you should start using heavier weights.

Progressive Overload

Progressive overloading is the key when it comes to making consistent gains in the gym. When we provide a stimulus like lifting weights to our body it reacts by adaptations by making our muscles bigger. Now when these muscles grow and you provide it with the same stimulus you did before they will maintain size but probably won't grow, now to make them even bigger we need to provide it with more stimulus than we did before. This is where Progressive Overload is helpful.

Its basically making your muscles work harder than what they are used to. Following are the ways to Progressively Overload and make your workouts more challenging :-

Let's understand this Concept with an Example, Suppose you lift 10kg for Bicep curl for 3 sets of 12 reps each, here are the ways in which you can apply the concept of Progressive Overloading to the exercise.

> **Increase the Weight**

The most common thing that a person can do is to simply increase the weight they are using, that would mean you can start using a 12kg Dumbbell instead of a 10kg.

> **Increase the Reps**

What you can also do is to increase the amount of reps you do. Instead of doing 12 reps you can try doing 15 reps.

> **Increase the Sets**

You can increase the number of sets you do for that exercise. Instead of doing 3 sets you can try doing 4.

> **Decrease the Rest time between Sets**

By resting less between a set you will do the same amount of work in shorter period of time. Let's say you rested 1 min between the sets before and now you only rest for 30 seconds between the sets.

Make sure you maintain good form during the whole Progressive Overloading period. Progressive Overloading mostly happen by itself, you don't have to force it. It is the result of you getting stronger. But it is still pushing yourself slightly. You can't be cheat curling to 15 reps and calling it progressive overloading, neither will lifting 12kg for reps using momentum will be considered as progressive overload.

So **Maintaining a standard /proper form** is crucial. Another major requirement for it is to keep a track of your workouts using a **Workout Logbook** so you can measure the progress or you will not be able to remember how much you lifted last time.

My Recommendation :-

You can either choose one way to overload or combine various ways to get to your goal. What i would suggest is to hit the upper limit of rep range say 15 reps with the 10kg dumbbell. Once you are able to do 15 reps for each set, you can add the weight to a bar. Of course adding the weight will cause your Rep range to drop, so now, lets say you are about to do 10 reps with 12kg now just work your way up to 15 reps again.

How Heavy should you lift?

One rep max- It is the maximum amount of weight that a person can lift for 1 Repetition.

For example let's say you can do maximum one rep (with Proper form) with 20kg dumbbell during a Bicep Curl,then,that 20 kg is your one rep max.

Training Types	Reps	% of 1RM	Goal
Strength	~ 1-6 (**Low**)	80-100 %	**Strength** and Muscle
Hypertrophy	~ 6-12 (**Moderate**)	60-80 %	**Muscle** and Strength
Endurance	~ 15 + (**High**)	< 60 %	**Endurance** and Muscle

How much Weight should you lift depends on what your Training Goal is?

Depends on what your Training Goal is?

- ➢ **Strength Training** is used by people who want to get stronger so they can prove their strength. This type of training is mostly used by Powerlifters.
- ➢ **Hypertrophy Training** is used by people who want to increase their muscle size. Most bodybuilders train for hypertrophy.
- ➢ **Endurance** means continuous supply of energy for a longer duration of time, for example in a sport like cycling a cyclist has to train himself more for endurance if he has take a part in a race.

Since every individual is different a single amount of weight can not be specified,hence we use **Percentage of your One Rep Max.**

Considering your main goal is to Build Muscle mass, i will suggest you to use Moderate Rep Ranges with load that is ~ 70% of your One Rep Max, Or in simple words, just pick up a weight that allows you to do not more than 10-15 reps with it.

Does that mean light weight (50%-70% of your One Rep Max,Weights you can do 15-20+ reps with) or super heavy weight(80%-100% of your One Rep Max,Weights you can do 1-9 reps with)does not build muscle?

The answer to that all rep ranges build muscles, but in my opinion that would not be the best way for you if you if want to grow maximum amount of muscles. However, You can incorporate the high reps and low reps ranges in your workouts if you really want to, but i would suggest you to stick to Moderate rep range for ¾ of your exercises .For the rest ¼ , you can try and test the low and high rep ranges.

You can use Lower reps on Compound movements to get stronger and Higher reps for isolation exercises to get that pump.

How long should you Rest between Sets?

Some say 30 seconds, some say at least 2 minutes, but i would suggest you to rest until you feel mentally ready to perform another quality set.

If you rest too little you won't be able to recover between the sets and push yourself hard in the next set and resting for too long we will make your workout sessions longer.

For small muscle group (Like Biceps, Triceps, Shoulders, Calves etc) and Isolation Movements 1-2 minute of rest is good and for Larger muscle groups (Chest, Back, Quads, Hamstrings, Glutes) and Compound Exercises 3-5 minute of rest should be fine.

How many Sets should you do ?

For smaller Muscle groups is 10-15 sets per week whereas for the bigger muscles 15-30 sets per week is recommended .As a beginner you might want to start at the lower side of the range. Now you might think that for smaller muscle group 10-15 sets per week is too little but keep in mind these muscle group also gets worked while training the larger muscle groups for example your Triceps gets trained when you train Chest and perform pushing movements and your Biceps gets trained when you do Back and perform pulling movements.

You should try not to do more than 10 sets per muscle group per workout session as the sets in the end will not be quality sets, as you would have tired your muscles already from the previous sets.

Frequency (How often should you workout?)

Frequency refers to the no of times you hit a muscle group. You can be hitting 20 sets per muscle group per week in two ways, you can either do those 20 sets for a muscle group in day or you can do 10 sets for that muscle 2 times a week. The second option will lead to more quality reps being performed in each set as your muscles fatigue after each subsequent set you perform. For each subsequent set you do the quality of reps will suffer slightly as you'd be tired from the previous sets.

Also let's say you do 20 sets of Biceps on Monday and then you train them again next Monday, but muscles takes only about 48-72 hrs or 2-3 days to recover. That leaves the remaining days go to waste where you could have trained and stimulated them again to grow, and with better quality sets.

But how can we train each muscle twice a week?

Thats when splits come into play. Usually people do **"The Bro Split "** under which they train only one Muscle group a day, and hit various muscle groups throughout the week.

For example:-

" The Bro Split "
Monday - Biceps
Tuesday - Chest
Wednesday - Back

Thursday - Legs
Friday - Shoulders
Saturday - Triceps
Sunday - Rest

Not saying that it doesn't result in gains for some individuals they might, but if you want to **Optimize** your Training Results you should train each body part at least 2x a week.

But how to do that do that? Following are some Split Routines that you can use.

FULL BODY SPLITS

In full body splits you train every muscle group in a single workout session ,then perform these sessions 3 times a week with at least one exercise per muscle group with and 48-72 hrs between each session. This split is most beginner friendly. Under this split every muscle is worked in moderation and mostly keeps you away from overtraining a particular muscle. This split keeps your volume low and frequency high, giving you good time to recover.

Tip-Train your lagging muscles at the beginning of the workout.

<u>Sample Full Body Split</u>

Monday - Full Body	Tuesday - Rest	Wednesday - Full Body	Thursday - Rest	Friday - Full Body	Saturday - Rest	Sunday - Rest

Bench press- 3-4 sets- 10-12 Reps
Squat- 3-4 sets -10-12 Reps

Deadlifts- 3-4 sets -10-12 Reps
Overhead Press- 3-4 sets -10-15 reps
Bicep Curls- 3-4 sets -12-15 reps
Tricep Extension- 3-4 sets – 12-15 reps

Upper-Lower Split

In the Upper Lower we train the whole body over a period of two days. We train the Upper Body one day (Arms,Chest,Legs,Shoulders,Back) and Lower body (Quads,Hamstrings,Glutes,Calves) another day, then we take a day off and then repeat it again. We perform at least 2 exercises for each muscle group every session with 2-4 sets each. This enables us to do more volume and allows Muscles we trained to rest and recover more.

Sample Upper-Lower Split

Monday	Tuesday	Wednesday	Thursday	Friday	Saturday	Sunday
-	-	-	-	-	-	-
Upper body	Lower body	Rest	Upper body	Lower Body	Rest	Rest

Upper Body	Lower Body
Bench Press – 3-4 sets – 10-12 Reps	**Squats** – 3-4 sets – 10 Reps
Cable Flys – 3-4 sets – 10-12 Reps	**Leg Extensions** – 3-4 sets – 10-12 Reps
Barbell Rows – 3-4 sets – 10-12 Reps	**Romanian Deadlift** – 3-4 sets – 10 Reps

Pull Ups – 3-4 sets – 10-15 Reps	**Hamstring Curls** – 3-4 sets – 10-12 Reps
Bicep Curls– 3-4 sets – 10-15 Reps	**Hip Thrusts** – 3-4 sets – 10-12 Reps
Tricep Extension– 3-4 sets – 10-15 Reps	**Standing/Seated calf raises** – 3-4 sets – 10-15 Reps
Skull Crushers – 3-4 sets – 10-15 Reps	
Overhead Press – 3-4 sets – 10-12 Reps	

Push-Pull-Legs Split

As we progress and our body get used to handling certain volume we can increase the volume by using the push-pull-legs split in which we train our entire body over the course of 3 days and then repeating it making it a 6 day workout split. You can combine muscle groups in different ways but most commonly on push day people train the muscles that are used for pushing like -Shoulders, Chest, Triceps and on pull days they train muscles that are used for pulling like Biceps & Back and then on leg day they do leg exercises. Recommended amount of exercises is at least 3 with 3-5 sets each.

Sample Push-Pull-Legs Split

Monday	Tuesday	Wednesday	Thursday	Friday	Saturday	Sunday
-	-	-	-	-	-	-
Push	Pull	Legs	Push	Pull	Legs	Rest

Push	Pull	Legs
Bench Press- 3-5 sets-10-12 Reps	**Deadlift-** 3-5 sets-10 Reps	**Squats-** 3-5 sets-10-12 Reps
Incline Bench Press- 3-5 sets - 10-12 Reps	**Bent Over Row-** 3-5 sets-10-12 Reps	**Romanian Deadlift –** 3-5 sets – 10 Reps
Dips- 3-5 sets-10-12 Reps	**Pull Ups-** 3-5 sets-10-12 Reps	**Leg Extensions –** 3-5 sets – 10-12 Reps
Overhead Press- 3-5 sets-10-12 Reps	**Bicep Curls-** 3-5 sets-10-12 Reps	**Hamstring Curls –** 3-5 sets – 10-12 Reps
Skull Crushers- 3-5 sets-10-12 Reps	**Hammer Curls-** 3-5 sets-10-12 Reps	**Hip Thrusts –** 3-5 sets – 10-12 Reps
Tricep Extension- 3-5 sets-10-12 Reps	**Face Pulls-** 3-5 sets-10-12 Reps	**Standing/Seated calf raises** – 3-5 sets – 10-15 Reps

You can choose whatever split fits your lifestyle the best and adjust the amount of sets and reps for yourself !

Recovery

Recovery is crucial if you want to actually build muscles. When you workout you break your muscles, you build your muscle when you give time to these muscles to recover and grow. If you don't allow your muscles to recover and keep training it continuously without rest you will reach a point of diminishing returns where more exercise won't result in more progress.

Following are the Tips to boost your Recovery :-

> **Proper Nutrition**

With your goal being muscle building you need to provide you body with proper nutrition. That means consuming the amount of calories and macros that your body Requires. The Protein we eat is used to build muscles so it is necessary for you to eat the required amount (0.8-1 gm/Lbs. Your Body Weight) to get most optimal results from your training. To recover your body needs energy so make sure you eat the amount of calories that your body requires.

> **Proper Sleep/Stress Management**

Sleep and Stress management are **crucial** when it comes to recovery, sadly these are the things most slept upon (no pun intended).Most people are so focused on Training and Dieting that they almost always ignore the importance of Sleep. A lot of Studies shows that 8-9 hr sleep is more optimal for both Fatloss and Muscle gain than the < 8 hr ones. If you have a very busy schedule do try to get the most amount of sleep possible.

Not Only recovery but sleeping also affects your training. If you don't get proper sleep you workouts will suffer next day and you won't be able to give your 100% in the gym, as you might feel tired.

Managing stress is crucial too because when we stress our body releases certain hormones(Like Cortisol) which slows down our ability to build muscle and lose fat.

> ➢ **Active/Passive Recovery**

Passive Recovery is when you are sedentary like sitting on couch, sleeping etc. Active recovery involves movements. Both of them are crucial but people often underestimate the effectiveness of active recovery .Active recovery involves really low intensity movements like yoga ,walking, swimming etc. What active recovery does is that it increases your blood flow to your muscles allowing nutrients to be transported to that muscle so your body can repair itself. My personal favourite will be just going for a simple 15-30 minute walk. Walking has also proven to improve your mood which might also help you to reduce Stress and it will also help you burn some calories.

> ➢ **Hydration**

When we work out our body loses water so it is necessary to keep yourself hydrated during the work out in order to maximize your performance in the gym. Even after work out make sure you are properly hydrated throughout the day as it improves recovery.

Supplements

Supplements are marketed heavily , so people often think that they can't build muscles without supplements, which is not true. There used to be a time when there were no supplements yet people achieved great physiques with just proper Diet and Training.

Following are the supplements that i would recommend. It's not mandatory to use these and you can make progress without them but you can use these, if you want, in addition to your diets and workouts for slightly better results.

> ➢ **Protein Powder**

We know by now that protein is really important to build muscles. Although i would suggest to consume most of your protein from whole foods but it might happen that you, sometimes don't have the time to eat food so in such cases you can use the Protein Powder as a supplement, as it is more convenient, in order to hit your daily Protein goals.

> ➢ **Creatine**

Creatine is one of the most researched supplement and has been proven to increase strength and muscle growth. If you want you can start consuming 3-5 gm/Day. It is known to cause slight water retention in some cases but you can try and test the results by yourself. Make sure you keep yourself hydrated when you consume Creatine to see some great results.